2hr Diet ™

Suzette Hay. BTchg.

Dedicated to my Creator,
my loving husband
and to my wonderful children.

CONTENTS

1 INTRODUCTION

Welcome to the 2hr Diet.

Congratulations on taking the first step to changing your life. Weight loss is not just about looking great but feeling great too. As you embark on this journey you will see physical change, you will gain a healthier body, you will experience changes to your self esteem and overall enhance your quality of life.

You may have tried many diets in the past but this one is different; you will not feel hungry on this diet. The 2hr Diet is not about eating less but eating the right foods, in the right quantities, at the right time. Dieters are never left hungry or feeling lethargic, in fact dieters often report they are eating more on the 2hr Diet.

With the 2hr Diet you can choose foods that you enjoy eating and leave the ones that you dislike. You can even get away with chocolate and eating out. You will lose weight and feel great!

Are you ready to embrace the new you?

2 METABOLISM &

WEIGHT LOSS

We all love to hate those people who seem to eat every naughty treat available, in copious amounts and still remain stick thin. In most cases these people have a high metabolic rate.

Metabolism is the many chemical processes which occur in the body as your body uses food energy to enable the body to function normally. The amount of kilojoules that your body burns is determined by your metabolism. Therefore if your metabolism is sluggish you will gain weight quicker than someone with a fast metabolism.

The rate of your metabolism or your metabolic rate can be restricted by a number of uncontrollable factors including:
1. Age - metabolism slows with age.
2. Hormonal issues.
3. Gender - as a rule men have faster metabolic rates than women....Ahhhh!
4. Genetic make-up.

Although you may have many of these uncontrollable factors, there are many ways to make your metabolism work efficiently and enable natural weight loss.

Two keys that are paramount in healthy, rapid weight loss are exercise and correct eating habits.

EXERCISE

Physical exercise causes the body to use up energy and hence burn kilojoules. Regular exercise will build up muscle mass and hence stimulate the body to burn kilojoules at a quicker rate, enabling the body to continue to burn fat well after the exercise is complete.

If you are anything like me, you will be time poor and possibly struggle with the thought of regular exercise but do not put the book down yet, there is hope! Although exercise will aid in quicker weight loss as well as providing other health benefits, I believe that 90% of weight loss or weight gain is a result of your eating habits. This is why you can lose weight simply by following the 2hr Diet program, using food to increase your metabolic rate.

CORRECT EATING HABITS

You can experience significant weight loss by simply controlling what you eat. It is not rocket science; if it does not go in your mouth, it will not go on your hips. This does not mean starving yourself, in fact quite the opposite. It is vital that you keep your metabolic rate high and you can do this by eating regularly (every two hours) and by eating certain foods in the right amounts.

Not eating enough food causes the body's metabolic rate to decrease, the body then stores food rather than metabolising it. Lack of food will also cause the muscle to break down, slowing the metabolic rate even further.

It takes energy for the body to digest food, so regular eating of low fat, low kilojoule foods will stimulate the body's metabolic rate and keep the body burning fat. After eating, your metabolic rate rises and continues to rise for approximately two hours as you digest your food.

The 2hr Diet is perfect for keeping your body working at burning kilojoules and breaking down fat. As you eat every two hours your metabolism is stimulated regularly causing natural weight loss.

3 HOW THE 2hr

DIET WORKS

Golden Rule:

Everyday you must eat 2 hourly over a 12 hour period, selecting foods from the food lists supplied.

Basic Rules:

1. You must eat seven times during any given day. If you choose to start eating at 7am, then your next snack or meal will be at 9am, then again at 11am, 1pm and so on.

2. You must have a glass of water every time you eat.

3. You can include up to 3 cups of tea or coffee with a small splash of skim milk and half a teaspoon of sugar (if required). You can have unlimited amounts of green or herbal teas.

4. One can of diet soft drink per day is allowed.

5. No condiments allowed (except salt and pepper) unless otherwise stated.

6. Remember that variety is the spice of life, when choosing foods you must select a variety from the lists, to ensure a balanced diet.

7. There are 3 lists of food items that you can choose from; Main Meal List, Snack List and Anytime Food List. For most people you will choose 3 items from the Main Meal List and 4 items from the Snack List for each day and you will consume them at 2 hour intervals. The Anytime Food List is a list of foods that you can eat anytime of the day and as much as you like.

8. If you are pregnant, breast feeding or have health issues, please consult your doctor before continuing.

You now have a basic understanding of how the 2hr Diet works, let's look at how you start.

IT'S AS EASY AS 1, 2, 3.

STEP 1: GOAL WEIGHT

Firstly you need to weigh yourself and record your starting weight. It would be beneficial to take some "before" photos as your body is about to change!

Then you need to decide on a realistic goal weight. Please examine the following table to assist you in this decision. Remember this is only a guide. You need to set a healthy weight that you feel you can reasonably achieve.

Determine how quickly you plan to lose your weight. For healthy weight loss that is easily maintained, I suggest you aim for 0.5 – 1.5kgs (1lb – 3lbs) of weight loss per week.

My Starting Weight _____

My Goal Weight _____

When I hope to achieve my Goal Weight ___ / ___ / _____

IDEAL WEIGHT RANGE

MENS CHART

Height		Small frame		Medium frame		Large frame	
cm	ft	kg	lb	kg	lb	kg	lb
165 - 167	5'5"	61-64	134-141	62 - 67	137-148	65 - 73	143-161
168 - 169	5'6"	62 - 64	137-141	63 - 69	139-152	66 - 74	146-163
170 - 172	5'7"	63 - 66	139-145	64 - 70	141-154	68 - 76	150-168
173 - 174	5'8"	64 - 67	141-148	66 - 71	146-156	69 - 78	152-172
175 - 177	5'9"	64 - 69	141-152	67 - 73	148-161	70 - 80	146-176
178 - 179	5'10"	65 - 70	143-154	69 - 74	152-163	72 - 82	152-172
180 - 182	5'11"	66 - 71	146-156	70 - 75	154-165	73 - 84	161-185
183 - 184	6'	68 - 73	150-161	71 - 77	156-170	74 - 85	163-187
185 - 187	6'1"	69 - 74	152-163	73 - 79	161-174	76 - 87	168-192
188 - 190	6'2"	70 - 76	154-168	74 - 81	163-179	78 - 89	172-196
191 - 192	6'3"	72 - 78	159-172	76 - 83	168-183	80 - 92	176-203
193 - 195	6'4"	74 - 80	163-176	78 - 85	172-187	82 - 94	181-207

WOMENS CHART

Height		Small frame		Medium frame		Large frame	
cm	Ft/in	kg	lb	kg	lb	kg	lb
155 - 157	5'1"	48 - 53	106-117	52 - 58	115-128	56 - 63	123-139
158 - 159	5'2"	49 - 54	108-119	53 - 59	117-130	58 - 64	128-141
160 - 162	5'3"	50 - 56	110-123	54 - 61	119-134	59 - 66	130-146
163 - 164	5'4"	51 - 57	112-126	56 - 62	123-137	66 - 68	146-150
165 - 167	5'5"	53 - 59	117-130	57 - 63	126-139	62 - 70	137-154
168 - 169	5'6"	54 - 60	119-132	59 - 65	130-143	63 - 72	139-159
170 - 172	5'7"	55 - 61	121-134	59 - 66	130-146	64 - 73	141-161
173 - 174	5'8"	57 - 63	126-139	61 - 68	134-150	66 - 75	146-165
175 - 177	5'9"	59 - 64	130-141	63 - 69	139-152	68 - 77	150-170
178 - 179	5'10"	59 - 65	130-143	64 - 70	141-154	68 - 78	150-172
180 - 182	5'11"	61 - 67	134-148	65 - 72	143-159	70 - 79	154-174
183 - 184	6'	62 - 68	137-150	67 - 73	148-161	71 - 81	157-179

STEP 2: LIST PROFILE

You now need to determine your List Profile. Based on your gender and weight you can determine how often you can choose foods from the Main and Snack lists. See the chart below to work out your List Profile.

LIST PROFILE CHART

WEIGHT		MALE	FEMALE
kg	lb		
<80	<177	4 Main + 3 Snack	3 Main + 4 Snack
80-120	177-265	4 Main + 3 Snack	4 Main + 3 Snack
>120	>265	5 Main + 2 Snack	4 Main + 3 Snack

STEP 3: DESIGN YOUR EATING PROGRAM

Design a workable program choosing items from the Main and Snack lists found in the following chapters. It does not matter what order your snack and mains are placed. See the example following.

SAMPLE PROGRAM: For a female weighing 73kg/161lb.

TIME	LIST	FOOD
6am	Main	2 eggs on 2 Toast
8am	Snack	Apple
10am	Snack	100g Low fat yogurt
12pm	Main	Ham & Salad Sandwich
2pm	Snack	2 Arrowroot biscuits
4pm	Snack	Banana
6pm	Main	Chicken breast & Vegetables

Construct your eating program for the next three days. It will not be long before you will not need to program; it will become a lifestyle. However strict planning in the beginning is vital for success.

MY 2hr DIET PROGRAM

DAY 1

TIME	LIST	FOOD

DAY 2

TIME	LIST	FOOD

DAY 3

TIME	LIST	FOOD

All the best! Now go for it!

4 MAIN MEAL LIST

BREAKFAST

- 2 French toast (See Recipe section)
- 2hr Diet omelette (See Recipe section)
- 2 pkts of Uncle Toby's instant porridge and 1 cup low fat milk
- 2 Toast and 4 tsp reduced fat butter and 4 tsp low joule jam
- 2 Toast (white/wholemeal/multigrain) and 2 eggs (not fried)
- 2 Weetbix and 1 cup of low fat milk
- Cornflakes 60g/2oz and ½ cup of low fat milk
- Coco pops 60g/2oz and ½ cup of low fat milk
- Nutri grain 60g/2oz and ½ cup of low fat milk
- Rice Bubbles 60g/2oz and ½ cup of low fat milk
- Special K 60g/2oz and ½ cup of low fat milk
- Sultana Bran 60g/2oz and ½ cup of low fat milk
- Sustain 60g/2oz and ½ cup of low fat milk

LUNCH

- 1 bread roll and banana
- 120g/4oz Skinless chicken breast and steamed vegetables from Anytime Food List
- 1 Variety sandwich (See Recipe section)
- 1 Weight Watchers satay chicken wrap
- 2hr Diet quiche and garden salad using items from Anytime Food List
- Turkish bread(15cm x 10cm) and tomato and 3 Tbs reduced fat cheese
- 2 Sushi rolls (No fried items)
- 2hr Diet vegetable frittata (See Recipe section)
- Nutra Life Carb Lite shake with skim milk and 1 banana
- Nutra Life Carb Lite shake with skim milk and 1 scoop low fat ice cream
- Hearty lamb soup (See Recipe section) and 1 bread roll
- 3 items from the Snack List
- Spicy chicken salad (See Recipe section)

DINNER

- Chicken, lamb or beef stir fry (See Recipe section)
- 1 Fish pan fried with oil spray/steamed/grilled and salad from Anytime Food List
- Lean Cuisine chicken and vegetable risotto frozen dinner
- Lean Cuisine thai green chicken curry with rice frozen dinner
- Lean Cuisine tuna bake frozen dinner
- Lean steak 125g/4.5oz and any vegetables or salad from Anytime Food List
- Vegetarian pasta (See Recipe section)
- Weight Watchers beef hot pot frozen dinner
- Weight Watchers chicken pesto spaghettini frozen dinner
- Weight Watchers cottage pie frozen dinner
- Weight Watchers creamy tomato gnocchi frozen dinner
- Weight Watchers peppered beef frozen dinner
- Weight Watchers thai chicken curry frozen dinner
- You'll love Coles lite beef hot pot frozen dinner
- Salmon cutlet 200g/7oz and salad from Anytime Food List
- Chips 97% fat free baked 100g/3.5oz and 1 egg (not fried) and lean steak 100g/3.5oz
- 2hr Diet pizza (See Recipe Section)

TAKEAWAY

- Hungry Jacks small french fries and salad (no dressing)
- KFC 1 Fried chicken piece
- KFC Small potato and gravy and small coleslaw
- McDonalds 1 cheeseburger and salad (no dressing)
- McDonalds 1 english muffin with jam or honey
- McDonalds 1 grilled chicken burger without sauce
- McDonalds 1 hash brown and 1 english muffin with butter
- McDonalds 1 junior burger
- Pizza 1 slice of vegetarian thin 'n crispy
- Pizza 1 slice of hawaiian thin 'n crispy
- Pizza 1 slice of supreme thin 'n crispy
- Red Rooster small potato and gravy and small coleslaw
- Red Rooster ¼ BBQ chicken leg
- Red Rooster 1 corn with butter and small coleslaw
- Red Rooster 2 skin free chicken pieces
- Red Rooster 5 chicken nuggets
- Subway any of the salads
- Subway any of the deli style sandwiches
- Subway turkey breast and ham 6 inch sub (no sauces)
- Subway ham 6 inch sub (no sauces)
- Subway roast beef 6 inch sub (no sauces)

5 SNACK LIST

BAKERY

- 1 Slice of bread and 2 tsp vegemite
- 1 Bakers Delight apricot delight
- 1 Bakers Delight coffee and date roll
- 1 Crumpet
- 1 Pikelet with low joule jam
- 1 Slice of bread and 1 tomato
- 1 Slice of bread and 2 tsp low joule jam
- Small turkish bread (credit card size) and ½ cup of salsa
- 2hr Diet scone (See Recipe section) and 2 tsp low joule jam
- 1 Soft citrus muffin (See Recipe section)
- Betty Crocker sweet rewards muffin mix, 1 muffin

BISCUITS AND CRACKERS

- 10 Rice crackers
- 1 Paradise Cottage biscuit
- 1 Rice cake and 1 Tbs low fat cottage cheese
- 2 Arrowroot biscuits
- 2 Corn thins and 1 Tbs low fat cottage cheese
- 2 Crackers and 2 tsp vegemite or 1 Tbs low joule jam
- 2 Girl Guide plain biscuits
- Arnotts Vita-Weat Grain snacks 20g/1oz pkt
- 2 Malt biscuits
- 2 Paradise Lites cookies
- 2 Weight Watchers biscuits
- 2 Arnotts rye cruskits and 2 tsp low joule jam
- 4 Water crackers and salsa

DAIRY AND DESSERT

- Low fat yogurt 100g/3.5oz
- 1 Egg (not fried)
- Fruche, light or whisp 125g/4.5oz tub
- Nestle Diet Strawberry Obsession
- Peters light and creamy vanilla slice
- Weight Watchers 145ml/5oz plain ice cream
- Weight Watchers 145ml/5oz cookies and cream ice cream
- Nestle diet creme caramel
- 1 Small scoop of low fat ice cream
- 1 Scoop of sorbet
- 1 Weight Watchers instant dessert
- 1 Weight Watchers instant mousse
- ½ Cup of low fat custard and low joule jelly
- Upside down cheesecake slice (See Recipe section)
- Soft serve in a cup (100ml/3oz – single serve)
- Baked custard supreme (See Recipe section)
- Banana split (See Recipe section)
- Pavlova (See Recipe section)
- Meringue Fruit Compote Nest (See Recipe Section)

DRIED FRUIT AND NUTS

- 10 Apple rings
- 10 Walnuts
- 1 Whole dried banana
- 1 Tbs Currants
- 1 Tbs Sultanas
- 1 Tbs Raisins
- 2 Figs
- 3 Apricots
- 5 Prunes
- 8 Almonds

FRUIT AND VEGETABLES

- 1 Apple
- 1 Carrot
- 1 Cup fruit salad
- 1 Cup pineapple
- 1 Custard apple
- 1 Mango
- 1 Orange
- 1 Pear
- 1 Punnet of strawberries
- 1 Small banana
- 2 Apricots
- 2 Cups of peas, carrots and sweet corn
- 2 Cups of watermelon
- 2 Figs
- 2 Kiwifruits
- 2 Mandarins
- 2 Plums
- 6 Lycees
- Edgell's four bean mix 125g/4.5oz
- SPC diced apricots 120g/4oz
- SPC fruit salad 120g/4oz
- SPC fruits in juice 120g/4oz two

OTHER

- Continental cup a soup spring vegetable
- Continental cup a soup pea and ham
- Continental cup a soup pumpkin
- Continental cup a soup tomato
- Weight Watchers can of tomato soup
- 1 Cup plain popcorn
- 1 Cappuccino on skim milk
- 10 Oysters
- Heinz spaghetti 130g/4.5oz
- Weight Watchers baked beans 130g/4.5oz
- 6 Mussels
- Wine 125ml/4oz
- 1 Uncle Tobys fruit fix
- 1 Nutritiously Tasti Fruitsies berry choc
- Tuna in springwater 95g/3oz
- Kelloggs LCMS rice bubble bar
- Uncle Tobys body wise bar berry fusion
- Fontelle fibre fix bar super berry
- Nutra Life Carb Lite shake (make with water)

SWEETS

- 5 Jube lollies
- 1 After dinner mint
- 1 Cup of Wendy's chocollo soft serve
- 1 Lamington finger
- 7 Jelly beans
- 2 Fantails
- 2 Licorice allsorts
- 4 Jaffas

TAKE AWAY

- Red Rooster 1 corn on cob
- Hungry Jacks salad (no dressing)
- KFC dinner roll
- KFC small mashed potato and gravy
- McDonalds salad (no dressing)
- Red Rooster 1 pineapple fritter

6 ANYTIME FOOD LIST

FRUIT & VEGETABLES

- Alfalfa sprouts
- Asparagus
- Bean sprouts
- Beans
- Beetroot
- Broccoli
- Cabbage
- Capsicum
- Carrot
- Cauliflower
- Celery
- Corn on the cob
- Cucumber
- Eggplant
- Grapefruit
- Leek
- Lettuce
- Mung bean sprouts
- Mushroom
- Onion

- Peas
- Pumpkin
- Radish
- Rhubarb
- Snow peas
- Spinach
- Swede
- Tomato
- Turnip
- Zucchini

EXTRAS

- Salsa
- Soy sauce
- Oyster sauce
- Fish sauce
- Worchester sauce
- Balsamic vinegar
- Soup (See Recipe section)
- Vegetable stir fry (See Recipe section)
- Wrigley's extra gum
- Low joule jelly

7 MAINTENANCE

Congratulations on losing weight!

Now that you have lost all your weight and feeling great, it's not time to celebrate with a family sized pizza, coke and half a mud cake. For those of us who have been over weight, it is easier for us to slip back into old habits and gradually gain the weight that we have worked so hard to lose.

So how do I keep the weight off? I'm glad you asked. Set your Target Weight. Your Target Weight is 3kg/6lb above your Goal Weight. For example, if your Goal Weight was 65kg/143lb with a 3kg/6lb buffer your Target Weight is 68kg/149lb.

So enjoy your new found confidence, new shape and your food but be sensible and remember to eat every 2 hours, drink water regularly and choose healthy food options in smaller portions. Monitor your weight weekly and if you reach your Target Weight then go back on the 2hr Diet until you are back to your Goal Weight. You will find that it will only take 1-2 weeks to get back to your Goal Weight again.

It's now time for you to write your own success story. Send us your "Before" and "After" photos and let us know how the 2hr Diet has worked for you. Email us at support@2hrdiet.com

We want to celebrate with you.

8 RECIPES

2hr DIET OMELETTE
Main

2 eggs
¼ cup skim milk
½ tomato diced
¼ small capsicum diced
1 diced mushroom
¼ onion diced
3 Tbs grated low fat cheese
oil spray

1. Spray lightly the pan with oil.
2. Saute onions.
3. Whisk milk and eggs, add to the pan.
4. When eggs are almost cook add tomato, mushroom and capsicum.
5. Sprinkle cheese on top.
6. Place under the grill until cheese melts. Serves 1.

2hr DIET PIZZA
Main

1 x 67g/2oz Bazaar wholemeal pita pocket
2 Tbs tomato paste
1 mushroom
½ tomato
¼ capsicum
¼ onion
¼ cup pineapple
50g/2oz of ham or one egg
3 Tbs grated reduced fat cheese

1. Spread pita pocket with tomato paste.
2. Wash and chop all toppings.
3. Add all ingredients on top of the pita bread with cheese last.
4. Cook in oven for 10 mins at 200°C/390°F.
Serves 1.

2hr DIET QUICHE
Main

6 eggs
¼ cup low fat milk
3 grated carrots
2 grated zucchini
1 diced onion
1 x 420g tin corn kernels
2 Tbs flour
100g/3.5oz grated low fat cheddar cheese
2 lean rashes bacon diced
oil spray

1. Sauté onion and bacon with a little oil spray until browned.
2. Combine eggs, milk and flour.
3. Add carrots, zucchini, corn and cooled bacon & onion to the egg mixture.
4. Mix well.
5. Spray pie dish with a small amount of oil spray, then add mixture.
6. Cook at 180°C/350°F for approximately 30 mins.

Serves 5

2hr DIET SCONES
Snack

1 cup plain flour
1 tsp baking powder
1/3 cup golden circle diet lemon and lime soda
1/3 cup low fat milk
low joule jam (2 tsp per scone)
salt to taste

1. Sift flour and baking powder.
2. Add salt, soda and milk.
3. Mix well.
4. Flour tray.
5. Roll into 6 scones and place on the tray.
6. Cook at 180°C/350°F for approximately 15 mins.

Serves 6

BAKED CUSTARD SUPREME
Snack

2½ cups skim milk
3 eggs
1 egg yolk
¼ cup castor sugar
2 tsp vanilla essence
nutmeg

1. Bring milk to the boil.
2. Whisk eggs, egg yolk, sugar and vanilla until just combined.
3. Gradually whisk hot milk into egg mixture.
4. Strain into shallow pie dish or 8 small dishes.
5. Sprinkle with nutmeg.
6. Place dish into a larger dish and pour boiling water into larger dish until it is halfway up the side of the custard dish.
7. Bake at 140°C/280°F for 45 mins or until it wobbles in the centre or the knife comes out clean.

Serves 8

BANANA SPLIT
Snack

½ banana
1 scoop low fat ice cream
1 wafer
1 Tbs low joule chocolate sauce

1. Split the ½ banana length ways and display in a banana split dish.
2. Place ice cream in between banana pieces.
3. Splash chocolate sauce over the ice cream and banana.
4. Cut the wafer on an angle making 2 triangles and display on top of ice cream.

Serves 1

CHICKEN/BEEF/LAMB STIR FRY
Main

120g/4oz chicken breast or lean beef or lean lamb
6 Tbs soy sauce
2 Tbs oyster sauce
2 Tbs fish sauce
2 carrots
1 zucchini
½ onion
10 snow peas
1 cup broccoli
oil spray
Any vegetables from Anytime Food List

1. Dice meat and brown in wok with a small amount of oil spray.
2. Cut and clean vegetables.
3. Add vegetables and heat.
4. Add soy sauce, oyster sauce and fish sauce and heat until vegetables and meat are coated in the sauce.

Serves 1

FRENCH TOAST
Main

1 slice bread
1 egg
2 Tbs low fat milk
1 Tbs sugar
cinnamon to taste
1 Tbs maple syrup
oil spray

1. Beat egg and combine with milk.
2. Dip bread into egg mixture.
3. Spray pan with small amount of oil.
4. Fry bread.
5. Top bread with sugar/cinnamon mix or maple syrup.

Serves 1

HEARTY LAMB SOUP
Main

1 lean lamb shank
½ Lt/17oz beef stock
½ Lt/17oz water
3 carrots
½ pumpkin
½ onion
1 potato
2 parsnips

1. Place lamb shank in a pot and cover with water, boil for approximately 2 hours or until the meat can be removed from the bone easily.
2. Wash, peel and dice all vegetables.
3. Place all vegetables, water and beef stock into a separate pot and boil until vegetables are soft.
4. Do not drain vegetables. Mash to preferred consistency.
5. Remove meat from shank and cut off any fat. Combine meat and vegetables and serve.

Serves 2

MERINGUE FRUIT COMPOTE NEST
Snack

2 egg whites
pinch of salt
½ cup caster sugar
2 tsp cornflour
1 tsp vinegar
¼ tsp vanilla essence
2 cups low fat yoghurt
1 cup chopped fruit (Strawberries, raspberries, kiwifruit, mango)
1 low joule jelly
oil spray

1. Beat egg whites and salt together until white peaks are formed.
2. Slowly add sugar whilst continually beating.
3. Add cornflour, vinegar and vanilla essence. Beat well.
4. Lightly spray oil on oven tray.
5. Divide mixture into 6 portions and shape into nests.
6. Cook in oven at 125°C/260°F for 1½ hours. Allow to cool.
7. Make jelly according to the instructions however reduce the water required to half of the suggested amount.
8. Once jelly is set, gently cut jelly into cubes.

9. Mix jelly, fruit and yoghurt together and divide into meringue nests.

Serves 6

PAVLOVA
Snack

4 egg whites
¼ tsp salt
1 cup caster sugar
4 tsp cornflour
2 tsp vinegar
½ tsp vanilla essence
1 cup Nestle D'lite yoghurt
6 strawberries
oil Spray

1. Line backing tray and spray with oil.
2. Beat the egg whites and salt until it forms soft peaks.
3. Gradually add sugar, beat well after each addition. Continue to beat until very stiff.
4. Add cornflour, vinegar and vanilla, beat well.
5. Pile mixture onto the tray and form pavlova.
6. Place in preheated oven at 125°C/260°F for 1½ hours.
7. When finished leave oven door closed until completely cold.
8. Top with yoghurt and sliced strawberries.

Serves 12

ROAST PUMPKIN SOUP
Snack

½ pumpkin
1 potato
1 parsnip
1 carrot
½ lt/17oz vegetable stock
oil spray
salt & pepper
2 Tbs milk

1. Peel and chop vegetables into small cubes.
2. Spray vegetables with oil spray and roast in the oven at 200°C/390°F until vegetables are soft and browned.
3. Put vegetables into a pot with vegetable stock and heat.
4. Blend soup, add milk, add salt & pepper and add more stock (if required) to give desired thickness.
5. To make this a meal, serve with 2 pieces of toast with 1 tsp of light margarine on each slice.

Serves 2

SOFT CITRUS MUFFINS
Snack

2 cups plain flour
2 tsp baking powder
½ tsp baking soda
½ cup low fat vanilla yoghurt
¼ cup lemon juice
¼ cup castor sugar
¼ cup orange juice
1 egg
oil spray
low joule jam

1. Sift flour, baking powder and baking soda and combine, set aside.
2. Mix together yoghurt, juices and sugar then add to flour mixture.
3. Lightly beat egg, add to mixture and mix until just combined.
4. Spray 12 cup muffin tin with oil and divide mixture evenly.
5. Cook for 15 mins on 200°C/390°F.
6. Serve with 2 tsp of low joule jam.

Serves 12

SPICY CHICKEN SALAD
Main

200g/7oz yellow string beans
½ tsp lime rind
1 Tbs lime juice
½ Tbs grated palm sugar
½ garlic clove
¼ Tbs peanut oil
¼ cup fresh mint
1 tsp sweet chilli sauce
½ Tbs fish sauce
200g/7oz cooked shredded chicken
¼ cup fresh coriander
½ punnet cherry tomatoes
½ small fresh red chilli

1. Trim beans and steam until tender.
2. Combine rind, juice, sugar, oil, mint, sweet chilli sauce and fish sauce.
3. Chop coriander, mint and chilli and halve tomatoes and add to sauce mixture.
4. Add beans and chicken to sauce mixture, toss and serve immediately.

Serves 2

UPSIDE DOWN CHEESECAKE SLICE
Snack

9 milk coffee biscuits
500g/1lb low fat cottage cheese
2 pkts lemon jelly
¼ cup of sugar
2 tsp orange rind
2 tsp lemon juice
strawberries

1. Dissolve jelly in 1 cup of boiling water and set aside to cool slightly.
2. Beat cottage cheese, sugar, lemon juice and rind.
3. Slowly add jelly mixture to cheese mixture, beating continuously.
4. Pour mixture into dish.
5. Place the biscuits on top of the mixture (biscuits should float) and refrigerate.
6. When set, cut into 9 slices and turn upside down.
7. Decorate with strawberries.

Serves 9

VARIETY SANDWICH
Main

2 slices of bread (white, wholemeal or multigrain)
lettuce
grated carrot
sliced tomato
sliced red onion (if desired)
sliced cucumber
1 Tbs low fat mayonnaise
Choose one of the following:
     50g/2oz ham
     50g/2oz turkey
     50g/2oz chicken (no skin)
     50g/2oz roast beef
     50g/2oz silver side
     1 boiled egg

1. Combine all ingredients between two slices of bread.
2. No butter or margarine allowed.

Serves 1

VEGETABLE FRITTATA
Main

6 eggs
¼ cup of low fat milk
3 Tbs grated low fat cheese
1 small sweet potato
¼ pumpkin
½ zucchini
1 cup broccoli
1 cup cauliflower
½ onion
1 tsp coriander
salt & pepper to taste
oil spray

1. Peel and slice vegetables.
2. Boil vegetables until just soft.
3. Spray dish with oil and layer vegetables.
5. Mix eggs, milk, coriander, salt, pepper.
6. Pour egg mixture over vegetables.
7. Sprinkle cheese on top.
8. Bake for approximately 30 mins at 180°C/350°F.

Serves 6

VEGETARIAN PASTA
Main

60g/2oz uncooked pasta
½ jar Coles brand pasta sauce
½ cup peas
½ cup corn
½ small capsicum diced
¼ onion diced
1 diced mushroom

1. Cook pasta as per packet instructions.
2. Sauté onions, capsicum and mushrooms.
3. Add pasta sauce to the onion mixture and heat.
4. Add peas, corn and pasta.
5. Heat well and serve.

Serves 1

VEGETABLE SOUP
Anytime Food

1 lt/34oz stock
¼ pumpkin
3 carrots
1 onion
Any other vegetable from Anytime Food List

1. Heat all ingredients in a pot until vegetables are soft.
2. Blend till preferred consistency.

Serves 2

VEGETABLE STIR FRY
Snack

6 Tbs soy sauce
2 Tbs oyster sauce
2 Tbs fish sauce
2 carrots
1 zucchini
½ onion
10 snow peas
1 cup broccoli
oil spray
Any vegetables from Anytime Food List

1. Cut and clean vegetables.
2. Spray wok with small amount of oil.
3. Heat all vegetables.
4. Add soy sauce, oyster sauce and fish sauce and heat until vegetables are coated in the sauce.
5. Check taste and add further sauces for own desired flavour.

Serves 1